GLUCOSE AND HEART HEALTH

Unraveling the Link between Blood Sugar and Cardiovascular Disease

By

Dr. Dimity Bertrand

Table of Contents
Introduction

Chapter 1

Glucose and Cardiovascular Disease

Chapter 2

Glucose Metabolism and Heart Disease

Chapter 3

Lifestyle Interventions for Optimizing Glucose and Cardiovascular Health

Chapter 4

Medical Interventions for Glucose Management and Cardiovascular Health

Chapter 5

Emerging Therapies for Glucose Management and Cardiovascular Health

Chapter 6

Lifestyle Interventions for Glucose Management and Cardiovascular Health

Chapter 7

Technology and Digital Solutions for Glucose Management and Cardiovascular Health

Chapter 8

Integrative Approaches for Glucose Management and Cardiovascular Health

Chapter 9

Behavioral Strategies for Sustaining Healthy Glucose Management and Cardiovascular Health

Chapter 10

Strategies for Long-Term Maintenance and Preventing Relapse

Introduction

elcome to "Glucose and Heart Health: Unraveling the Link between Blood Sugar and Cardiovascular Disease."

In this book, we delve into the fascinating connection between glucose levels and one of the most prevalent health concerns of our time: cardiovascular disease.

Heart disease remains the leading cause of death worldwide, and its prevention and management are critical for improving global health outcomes.

While many factors contribute to the development of cardiovascular disease, emerging research has shed light on the significant role of glucose metabolism in its pathogenesis.

This book serves as a comprehensive guide to help you understand the intricate relationship between glucose and heart health.

We will explore the latest scientific findings and provide practical insights into how managing blood sugar levels can positively impact cardiovascular health.

In the following chapters, we will embark on an enlightening journey, examining the various mechanisms by which glucose affects the cardiovascular system.

We will uncover the intricate interplay between glucose metabolism, insulin resistance, inflammation, and lipid profiles and how these factors contribute to the development of heart disease.

Furthermore, we will discuss the impact of dietary choices and lifestyle habits on blood sugar regulation and cardiovascular health.

From exploring the effects of refined sugars and processed foods to understanding the benefits of physical activity and stress management, we will provide you with actionable strategies for maintaining optimal glucose levels and promoting a healthy heart.

Throughout this book, we will also address the unique challenges faced by individuals with diabetes or pre-diabetes, as they are particularly vulnerable to heart disease.

We will outline evidence-based approaches to managing blood sugar in these populations and offer practical guidance for preventing and managing cardiovascular complications.

Finally, we will touch upon the exciting developments in medical technology and pharmacotherapy, highlighting how advances in glucose monitoring and insulin therapies can benefit individuals at risk of cardiovascular disease.

Whether you are a healthcare professional, a patient seeking to optimize your heart health, or someone interested in the fascinating connection between glucose and cardiovascular disease, this book will provide you with a solid foundation of knowledge, practical strategies, and empowering insights.

We hope that "Glucose and Heart Health: Unraveling the Link between Blood Sugar and Cardiovascular Disease" will not only broaden your understanding of the intricate relationship between glucose and cardiovascular health but also inspire you to take proactive steps towards a heart-healthy lifestyle.

Let's embark on this enlightening journey together and unlock the secrets to a thriving heart and a fulfilling life.

Chapter One

Glucose and Cardiovascular Disease

Cardiovascular disease (CVD) is a widespread health concern, responsible for significant morbidity and mortality worldwide.

It encompasses a range of conditions, including coronary artery disease, heart failure, and stroke, which collectively pose a considerable burden on individuals, families, and healthcare systems.

While the causes of CVD are multifactorial, recent research has shed light on the crucial role of glucose metabolism in the development and progression of heart disease.

In this chapter, we will explore the intricate relationship between glucose and cardiovascular health, providing a foundation for understanding the subsequent chapters of this book.

Understanding the prevalence and impact of cardiovascular disease

Cardiovascular disease remains a leading cause of death globally, with millions of lives affected each year.

Factors such as sedentary lifestyles, unhealthy dietary patterns, smoking, and stress contribute to the increasing incidence of CVD.

It is essential to recognize the significance of this health issue and the need for effective preventive strategies and management approaches.

Overview of the role of glucose metabolism in heart health

Glucose, a vital source of energy for the body, plays a pivotal role in various physiological processes.

It serves as the primary fuel for the heart, enabling its continuous pumping action.

However, disturbances in glucose metabolism, such as insulin resistance and impaired glucose tolerance, can have detrimental effects on cardiovascular health.

These metabolic dysregulations may lead to the development of diabetes, a major risk factor for heart disease.

Understanding the intricate relationship between glucose metabolism and heart health is crucial for preventing and managing CVD effectively.

Significance of blood sugar regulation for cardiovascular health.

Maintaining optimal blood sugar levels is essential for cardiovascular health.

Chronically elevated blood glucose levels can lead to the formation of advanced glycation end products (AGEs), which contribute to inflammation, oxidative stress, and damage to blood vessels.

This vascular damage can result in atherosclerosis, the buildup of plaque in the arteries, increasing the risk of heart attacks and strokes.

On the other hand, episodes of low blood sugar (hypoglycemia) can lead to adverse cardiovascular events due to the stress placed on the heart.

Achieving and maintaining a balance in blood sugar regulation is paramount for preserving heart health.

Furthermore, glucose metabolism influences several other processes that impact cardiovascular health.

Insulin, a hormone involved in glucose regulation, has additional effects on blood vessel function, lipid metabolism, and inflammation.

Dysfunctions in these areas can contribute to the development and progression of CVD.

Key points covered in Chapter 1

- ✓ Cardiovascular disease is a significant global health concern.
- ✓ Factors such as lifestyle choices and genetic predisposition contribute to the development of CVD.
- ✓ Glucose metabolism plays a critical role in cardiovascular health.
- ✓ Disturbances in glucose metabolism can lead to insulin resistance and diabetes, increasing the risk of heart disease.

✓ Optimal blood sugar control is essential for preventing vascular damage and reducing the risk of heart attacks and strokes.

✓ Glucose metabolism influences various processes, including blood vessel function, lipid metabolism, and inflammation, which impact cardiovascular health.

By establishing this groundwork, Chapter 1 sets the stage for a comprehensive exploration of the intricate relationship between glucose and cardiovascular disease.

It highlights the importance of glucose metabolism in heart health and its subsequent impact on cardiovascular outcomes.

With this knowledge in hand, readers can embark on an enlightening journey to uncover the various mechanisms, lifestyle interventions, and treatment strategies that promote a healthy heart and optimal glucose control.

The subsequent chapters will delve deeper into these topics, providing practical insights and evidence-based approaches for managing blood sugar and improving cardiovascular health.

Chapter Two

Glucose Metabolism and Heart Disease

In this chapter, we will delve deeper into the intricate relationship between glucose metabolism and heart disease.

We will explore the mechanisms by which disturbances in glucose metabolism, such as insulin resistance and impaired glucose tolerance, contribute to the development and progression of cardiovascular disease.

Understanding these mechanisms is essential for designing effective strategies to prevent and manage heart disease.

Exploring the mechanisms linking glucose metabolism and cardiovascular disease

1. Insulin Resistance

Insulin resistance plays a central role in the connection between glucose metabolism and heart disease.

Insulin is a hormone produced by the pancreas that helps regulate glucose levels in the bloodstream.

However, in individuals with insulin resistance, the body's cells become less responsive to insulin's actions, resulting in reduced glucose uptake.

As a consequence, blood sugar levels remain elevated, leading to a cascade of metabolic disturbances that increase the risk of cardiovascular disease.

Insulin resistance promotes the release of pro-inflammatory cytokines, triggers oxidative stress, and alters lipid metabolism, all of which contribute to the development of atherosclerosis and cardiovascular complications.

2. Inflammation and Oxidative Stress

Dysregulated glucose metabolism contributes to chronic low-grade inflammation and oxidative stress, which play pivotal roles in the development of cardiovascular disease.

Elevated blood glucose levels activate inflammatory pathways, leading to the production of pro-inflammatory cytokines and the recruitment of immune cells to the arterial walls.

In turn, these inflammatory processes contribute to endothelial dysfunction and the formation of atherosclerotic plaques.

Oxidative stress, resulting from an imbalance between the production of reactive oxygen species and antioxidant defenses, further exacerbates the inflammatory response, damages blood vessels, and promotes atherosclerosis.

3. Endothelial Dysfunction

The endothelium, a thin layer of cells that lines the inner surface of blood vessels, plays a crucial role in maintaining vascular health.

In conditions of impaired glucose metabolism, such as insulin resistance and hyperglycemia, endothelial dysfunction occurs.

This dysfunction is characterized by reduced nitric oxide production, increased oxidative stress, inflammation, and impaired vasodilation.

Endothelial dysfunction contributes to the development of hypertension, accelerates the progression of atherosclerosis, and promotes the formation of blood clots, all of which increase the risk of cardiovascular events.

4. Lipid Metabolism

Glucose metabolism and lipid metabolism are intricately linked, and disturbances in one can impact the other.

Insulin resistance and impaired glucose tolerance disrupt lipid metabolism, leading to dyslipidemia, characterized by elevated levels of triglycerides and LDL cholesterol and decreased levels of HDL cholesterol.

Dyslipidemia contributes to the formation of atherosclerotic plaques by promoting the accumulation of cholesterol in the arterial walls.

It also affects the balance between pro-inflammatory and anti-inflammatory lipid profiles, further fueling the inflammatory response and the development of cardiovascular disease.

5. Hyperglycemia and Advanced Glycation End Products (AGEs)

Prolonged exposure to high blood glucose levels, as seen in diabetes or poorly controlled blood sugar, leads to the formation of advanced glycation end products (AGEs).

AGEs are formed when glucose molecules attach to proteins, altering their structure and function.

These modified proteins can activate receptors called RAGEs (receptors for advanced glycation end products), triggering an inflammatory response and oxidative stress.

AGEs contribute to endothelial dysfunction, inflammation, and oxidative stress, accelerating the progression of atherosclerosis and cardiovascular disease.

Additionally, AGEs can promote platelet activation and contribute to thrombosis, further increasing the risk of cardiovascular events.

Understanding these mechanisms helps us recognize the intricate connections between glucose metabolism and heart disease.

By addressing disturbances in glucose metabolism and mitigating their effects on these mechanisms, we can potentially prevent or slow the progression of cardiovascular disease.

Key points covered in Chapter 2

✓ Insulin resistance is a central player in the connection between glucose metabolism and heart disease.

✓ Dysregulated glucose metabolism contributes to chronic inflammation and oxidative stress, promoting the formation of atherosclerotic plaques.

✓ Endothelial dysfunction, characterized by impaired nitric oxide production and increased oxidative stress, contributes to the progression of heart disease.

✓ Disturbances in glucose metabolism can lead to dyslipidemia, increasing the risk of atherosclerosis.

✓ Hyperglycemia and advanced glycation end products (AGEs) accelerate the progression of atherosclerosis and cardiovascular disease.

By examining these mechanisms, we gain a deeper understanding of how disturbances in glucose metabolism contribute to the development and progression of heart disease.

Armed with this knowledge, we can explore targeted interventions and treatment strategies in subsequent chapters to effectively manage glucose levels and mitigate the impact on cardiovascular health.

The forthcoming chapters will delve into lifestyle modifications, medical interventions, and emerging therapies aimed at optimizing glucose metabolism and promoting heart health.

Chapter Three

Lifestyle Interventions for Optimizing Glucose and Cardiovascular Health

Building upon that foundation, Chapter 3 will delve into the role of lifestyle interventions in optimizing glucose metabolism and promoting cardiovascular health.

Lifestyle modifications, including dietary changes, regular physical activity, weight management, stress reduction, and the avoidance of harmful habits, can have a significant impact on glucose control and the prevention of heart disease.

Understanding and implementing these interventions can empower individuals to take control of their health and improve their overall well-being.

1. Dietary Modifications

Diet plays a critical role in glucose metabolism and cardiovascular health. Specific dietary modifications that can optimize glucose control and reduce the risk of heart disease include:

a. Glycemic Load Management

The glycemic load takes into account both the quality and quantity of carbohydrates consumed. By focusing on foods with a lower glycemic load, such as whole grains, legumes, and non-starchy vegetables, individuals can minimize blood sugar spikes and promote more stable glucose levels.

b. Portion Control

Controlling portion sizes is essential for maintaining balanced blood sugar levels.

By being mindful of portion sizes and avoiding excessive calorie intake, individuals can better manage their glucose metabolism and promote weight management.

c. Nutrient-Rich Choices

Opting for nutrient-dense foods, such as fruits, vegetables, lean proteins, and healthy fats, provides essential vitamins, minerals, and antioxidants that support glucose control and cardiovascular health.

These choices also contribute to overall nutritional balance and well-being.

2. Regular Physical Activity

Engaging in regular physical activity is vital for optimizing glucose metabolism and cardiovascular health.

Exercise has multiple benefits, including:

a. Improved Insulin Sensitivity

Physical activity enhances insulin sensitivity, allowing cells to efficiently take up glucose from the bloodstream.

This helps regulate blood sugar levels and reduces the risk of insulin resistance.

b. Weight Management

Physical activity contributes to weight management by increasing energy expenditure and promoting the maintenance of lean muscle mass.

By maintaining a healthy weight, individuals can improve glucose control and reduce the risk of heart disease.

c. Cardiovascular Fitness

Regular aerobic exercise, such as brisk walking, jogging, cycling, or swimming, strengthens the heart and improves cardiovascular fitness.

This leads to improved blood circulation, better oxygen delivery, and a reduced risk of heart disease.

3. Weight Management

Maintaining a healthy weight is crucial for optimizing glucose metabolism and cardiovascular health.

Excess body weight, particularly visceral adiposity (abdominal fat), is associated with insulin resistance, dyslipidemia, inflammation, and an increased risk of heart disease. Strategies for weight management include:

a. Calorie Control

Consuming an appropriate number of calories based on individual energy needs is important for maintaining a healthy weight.

This can be achieved through portion control, mindful eating, and balancing energy intake with physical activity.

b. Balanced Diet

A balanced and nutrient-rich diet supports weight management by providing essential nutrients while minimizing excessive calorie intake.

Emphasizing whole, unprocessed foods and limiting added sugars and unhealthy fats can contribute to weight loss or maintenance.

c. Behavior Modification

Adopting healthy eating habits and lifestyle behaviors is crucial for long-term weight management.

Strategies such as mindful eating, keeping a food diary, seeking social support, and addressing emotional triggers for overeating can all contribute to successful weight management.

4-Stress Reduction

Chronic stress can have negative effects on glucose metabolism and cardiovascular health.

Implementing stress reduction techniques can help improve glucose control and overall well-being.

Some strategies include:

a. Relaxation Techniques

Techniques such as deep breathing exercises, progressive muscle relaxation, and meditation can help reduce stress levels and promote a sense of calm and relaxation.

b. Physical Activity

Engaging in regular physical activity not only improves physical fitness but also acts as a stress reliever.

Exercise stimulates the release of endorphins, which are natural mood boosters and stress reducers.

c. Adequate Sleep

Prioritizing quality sleep is essential for stress reduction. Lack of sleep or poor sleep quality can increase stress levels and negatively impact glucose control.

Aim for 7-8 hours of uninterrupted sleep each night.

5-Avoidance of Harmful Habits

Certain habits can have detrimental effects on glucose metabolism and cardiovascular health.

It is important to avoid or limit the following:

a. Smoking

Smoking is a significant risk factor for both cardiovascular disease and insulin resistance. Quitting smoking can lead to improvements in insulin sensitivity and cardiovascular health.

b. Excessive Alcohol Consumption

Heavy alcohol intake can disrupt glucose regulation, contribute to liver dysfunction, and increase the risk of insulin resistance and heart disease.

Moderation is key, and individuals should adhere to the recommended limits for alcohol consumption.

By implementing these lifestyle interventions, individuals can take proactive steps to optimize their glucose control and promote cardiovascular health.

Remember, small changes can have a significant impact over time.

The forthcoming chapters will explore medical interventions and emerging therapies that complement lifestyle changes, providing a comprehensive approach to managing glucose metabolism and preventing heart disease.

Chapter Four

Medical Interventions for Glucose Management and Cardiovascular Health

In this chapter, we will explore various medical interventions available for individuals with disturbances in glucose metabolism and an increased risk of cardiovascular disease.

These interventions, ranging from pharmacological treatments to surgical procedures, aim to improve glucose control, manage risk factors, and reduce the incidence of cardiovascular complications.

Understanding these medical interventions can provide individuals with additional tools to optimize their health and reduce the impact of glucose-related cardiovascular risks.

1. Medications for Glucose Control

Several medications are available to help manage glucose levels in individuals with diabetes or impaired glucose tolerance.

These medications work through different mechanisms to enhance insulin sensitivity, promote insulin secretion, or reduce glucose production.

Commonly prescribed medications include:

a. Metformin

Metformin is a first-line medication for type 2 diabetes that improves insulin sensitivity and reduces glucose production in the liver.

It is often prescribed as an initial treatment and can be used in combination with other medications.

b. Sulfonylureas

These medications stimulate insulin secretion from pancreatic beta cells, increasing insulin levels in the bloodstream.

They are commonly prescribed for type 2 diabetes but can carry a risk of hypoglycemia.

c. DPP-4 Inhibitors

Dipeptidyl peptidase-4 (DPP-4) inhibitors enhance the action of cretin hormones, which help regulate glucose levels by increasing insulin secretion and reducing glucagon release.

These medications are typically well-tolerated and have a lower risk of hypoglycemia.

d. SGLT2 Inhibitors

Sodium-glucose co-transporter 2 (SGLT2) inhibitors work by reducing glucose reabsorption in the kidneys, leading to increased urinary glucose excretion.

They also have additional benefits for cardiovascular outcomes, such as reducing the risk of heart failure and cardiovascular events.

2. Blood Pressure Management

Hypertension, or high blood pressure, is a common risk factor for cardiovascular disease.

Individuals with disturbances in glucose metabolism often have an increased risk of hypertension.

Medications for blood pressure management are essential for optimizing cardiovascular health.

Commonly prescribed medications include:

a. Angiotensin-Converting Enzyme (ACE) Inhibitors

ACE inhibitors reduce the production of angiotensin II, a hormone that constricts blood vessels and increases blood pressure.

By blocking this hormone, ACE inhibitors help lower blood pressure and protect against cardiovascular complications.

b. Angiotensin II Receptor Blockers (ARBs)

ARBs work by blocking the action of angiotensin II at its receptors, leading to blood vessel relaxation and reduced blood pressure.

They are often prescribed as an alternative to ACE inhibitors, particularly for individuals who may experience side effects from ACE inhibitors.

c. Calcium Channel Blockers

Calcium channel blockers relax and widen blood vessels by inhibiting calcium influx into smooth muscle cells.

This helps lower blood pressure and improve blood flow to the heart.

d. Diuretics

Diuretics increase urine production, thereby reducing fluid volume in the body and lowering blood pressure.

They are commonly used as part of combination therapy for hypertension management.

3. Lipid Management

Disturbances in glucose metabolism often coincide with dyslipidemia, which is characterized by elevated levels of LDL cholesterol and triglycerides and reduced levels of HDL cholesterol.

Medications for lipid management are crucial for reducing the risk of atherosclerosis and cardiovascular events.

Commonly prescribed medications include:

a. Statins

Statins are widely used to lower LDL cholesterol levels by inhibiting an enzyme involved in cholesterol synthesis.

They also have additional benefits for stabilizing atherosclerotic plaques and reducing inflammation.

b. Fibrates

Fibrates primarily target elevated triglyceride levels and can also increase HDL cholesterol levels.

They work by activating enzymes involved in triglyceride breakdown and reducing triglyceride synthesis.

c. Ezetimibe

Ezetimibe reduces LDL cholesterol absorption from the intestine, thereby lowering LDL cholesterol levels.

It is often used in combination with statins for individuals who require further LDL cholesterol reduction.

d. PCSK9 Inhibitors

PCSK9 inhibitors are a newer class of medications that lower LDL cholesterol levels by inhibiting a protein involved in its degradation.

They are typically reserved for individuals with very high LDL cholesterol or who cannot tolerate statins.

4. Antiplatelet Therapy

Individuals with disturbances in glucose metabolism are at increased risk of cardiovascular events such as heart attacks and strokes.

Antiplatelet therapy is often prescribed to reduce the risk of blood clot formation.

Commonly used antiplatelet medications include:

a. Aspirin

Aspirin inhibits platelet aggregation and reduces the formation of blood clots.

It is commonly prescribed for individuals at high risk of cardiovascular events.

b. P2Y12 Inhibitors

P2Y12 inhibitors, such as clopidogrel, ticagrelor, and prasugrel, block a receptor on platelets, reducing their ability to aggregate.

They are often prescribed in combination with aspirin for individuals with acute coronary syndromes or those who have undergone coronary stenting.

5. Surgical Interventions

In certain cases, surgical interventions may be necessary to manage cardiovascular risks associated with disturbances in glucose metabolism.

These interventions include:

a. Coronary Artery Bypass Grafting (CABG)

CABG involves bypassing blocked or narrowed coronary arteries using blood vessels from other parts of the body.

This surgical procedure restores blood flow to the heart, reducing the risk of heart attacks and improving cardiovascular outcomes.

b. Percutaneous Coronary Intervention (PCI)

PCI, also known as angioplasty, involves inserting a balloon-tipped catheter into narrowed or blocked coronary arteries.

The balloon is inflated to widen the artery, and a stent may be placed to maintain blood flow.

This procedure is often performed in individuals with coronary artery disease to alleviate symptoms and reduce the risk of cardiovascular events.

c. Bariatric Surgery

Bariatric surgery may be considered for individuals with severe obesity and associated metabolic conditions, such as diabetes and cardiovascular risks.

These surgical procedures promote weight loss and can significantly improve glucose control and cardiovascular outcomes.

By incorporating these medical interventions alongside lifestyle modifications, individuals can further optimize their glucose control and reduce the risk of cardiovascular complications.

However, it is important to note that medical interventions should always be prescribed and overseen by healthcare professionals who consider individual needs, preferences, and potential side effects.

6. Diabetes Medications for Cardiovascular Protection

In addition to medications specifically targeting glucose control, there are newer classes of diabetes medications that have shown significant cardiovascular benefits.

These medications go beyond glucose management and have demonstrated the ability to reduce the risk of cardiovascular events.

Some notable classes include:

a. GLP-1 Receptor Agonists

GLP-1 receptor agonists are injectable medications that mimic the action of glucagon-like peptide-1, an incretin hormone involved in glucose regulation.

In addition to improving glucose control, GLP-1 receptor agonists have been shown to reduce the risk of heart attacks, strokes, and cardiovascular mortality.

They also promote weight loss and have beneficial effects on blood pressure and lipid profiles.

b. SGLT2 Inhibitors

We mentioned SGLT2 inhibitors earlier as medications for glucose control, but they also offer significant cardiovascular benefits.

These medications not only lower blood glucose levels but have been shown to reduce the risk of heart failure hospitalizations, cardiovascular death, and kidney disease progression.

SGLT2 inhibitors work by increasing urinary glucose excretion and have additional effects on reducing blood pressure and improving arterial function.

7. Hypoglycemia Management

For individuals using glucose-lowering medications, the risk of hypoglycemia (low blood sugar) can be a concern.

Hypoglycemia can have serious consequences and may impact cardiovascular health.

Therefore, it is important to have strategies in place to prevent and manage hypoglycemic episodes.

Some considerations include:

a. Individualized Glucose Targets

Setting appropriate glucose targets for each individual is crucial to avoiding excessive glucose lowering and the associated risk of hypoglycemia.

Healthcare providers work with patients to establish personalized goals based on factors such as age, health status, and overall cardiovascular risk.

b. Medication Adjustments

Dosage adjustments or changes in medication regimens may be necessary to minimize the risk of hypoglycemia while maintaining optimal glucose control.

This may involve reducing the dose of certain medications or switching to alternative agents with a lower risk of hypoglycemia.

c. Regular Blood Glucose Monitoring

Regular self-monitoring of blood glucose levels allows individuals to track their glucose patterns and identify any potential episodes of hypoglycemia.

This enables timely intervention and adjustment of medications or lifestyle factors as needed.

8. Patient Education and Shared Decision-Making

When considering medical interventions for glucose management and cardiovascular health, patient education and shared decision-making play a vital role.

Healthcare providers should engage in comprehensive discussions with individuals to ensure they have a clear understanding of the benefits, risks, and potential side effects of each intervention.

This empowers individuals to actively participate in their care and make informed decisions that align with their preferences and goals.

It is important to note that medical interventions should always be prescribed and monitored by healthcare professionals who consider the individual's unique circumstances, medical history, and potential interactions with other medications.

Close collaboration between individuals and healthcare providers ensures the most appropriate treatment plan is established to optimize glucose control and cardiovascular health.

In the subsequent chapters, we will explore emerging therapies and advancements in medical interventions for glucose management and cardiovascular health.

These new developments offer exciting prospects for further improving outcomes and reducing the burden of cardiovascular disease in individuals with disturbances in glucose metabolism.

Chapter Five

Emerging Therapies for Glucose Management and Cardiovascular Health

n this Chapter, we explore the latest developments and promising approaches that show potential for optimizing glucose control, reducing cardiovascular risks, and improving overall health outcomes.

These emerging therapies go beyond traditional pharmacological interventions and encompass innovative techniques and technologies that hold great promise for individuals with disturbances in glucose metabolism.

1. Precision Medicine

Precision medicine is an evolving field that aims to tailor medical interventions to an individual's unique characteristics, such as genetic makeup, lifestyle, and environmental factors.

By considering these factors, healthcare providers can personalize treatment plans and optimize glucose management and cardiovascular health outcomes. Key components of precision medicine include:

a. Genetic Testing

Genetic testing enables the identification of specific genetic variations that may impact an individual's response to medications and their susceptibility to certain diseases. Understanding an individual's genetic profile can aid in selecting the most effective medications and dosages.

b. Pharmacogenomics

Pharmacogenomics examines how an individual's genetic makeup influences their response to medications.

By analyzing genetic variations, healthcare providers can identify potential drug interactions, predict treatment outcomes, and select medications that are most likely to be effective and safe for a particular individual.

c. Personalized Nutritional Strategies

Precision medicine also extends to personalized nutritional strategies.

Understanding an individual's metabolic profile and genetic predispositions can guide the development of personalized dietary recommendations, ensuring optimal glucose control and cardiovascular health.

2. Continuous Glucose Monitoring (CGM)

Continuous glucose monitoring is a technology that allows individuals to track their glucose levels in real time throughout the day and night.

CGM systems use a tiny sensor inserted under the skin to measure glucose levels in the interstitial fluid.

This data is wirelessly transmitted to a device that displays the glucose readings and provides trends and alerts.

CGM offers several advantages:

a. Real-Time Glucose Monitoring

CGM provides individuals with immediate feedback on their glucose levels, enabling them to make timely adjustments to their diet, physical activity, and medication regimen.

b. Trend Analysis

CGM systems provide trend arrows that indicate the direction and rate of glucose changes.

This allows individuals to identify patterns and adjust their management strategies accordingly.

c. Hypoglycemia and Hyperglycemia Alerts

CGM devices can be programmed to send alerts when glucose levels are too high or too low, helping individuals prevent or manage potentially dangerous episodes.

d. Data Sharing

Many CGM systems allow individuals to share their glucose data with healthcare providers or caregivers.

This facilitates remote monitoring and collaborative management.

3. Artificial Pancreas Systems

Artificial pancreas systems, also known as closed-loop systems or hybrid closed-loop systems, combine continuous glucose monitoring with automated insulin delivery.

These systems use algorithms to analyze glucose data and adjust insulin delivery through an insulin pump.

The aim is to mimic the function of a healthy pancreas by continuously monitoring glucose levels and delivering the appropriate amount of insulin.

Key features of artificial pancreas systems include:

a. Automation

Artificial pancreas systems automate insulin delivery, reducing the need for frequent manual injections or adjustments.

b. Improved Glucose Control

By continuously monitoring glucose levels and adjusting insulin delivery in real-time, artificial pancreas systems can help individuals achieve better glucose control, minimizing both hyperglycemic and hypoglycemic episodes.

c. Reduced Burden

These systems can significantly reduce the burden of diabetes management by taking on some of the decision-making and adjustment tasks.

4. Stem Cell Therapy

Stem cell therapy holds promise for regenerative medicine and may offer new avenues for glucose management and cardiovascular health.

Stem cells have the potential to differentiate into various cell types, including insulin-producing cells or cells that repair damaged tissues.

Although still in the experimental stage, stem cell therapy shows potential for:

a. Regenerating Beta Cells

Stem cells may be used to generate insulin-producing beta cells that can replace damaged or dysfunctional cells in individuals with diabetes.

This approach could restore normal glucose metabolism and reduce the need for exogenous insulin.

b. Tissue Repair and Regeneration

Stem cells can repair damaged tissues and improve vascular function, which is crucial for cardiovascular health.

By promoting tissue repair and regeneration, stem cell therapy may reduce the risk of complications associated with disturbances in glucose metabolism.

c. Immunomodulation

Stem cells can also modulate the immune system, potentially preventing the autoimmune destruction of beta cells in type 1 diabetes or mitigating chronic inflammation associated with insulin resistance and cardiovascular disease.

5. Telemedicine and Digital Health Solutions

Advancements in telemedicine and digital health solutions have transformed the way healthcare is delivered, especially in the fields of glucose management and cardiovascular health.

These technologies offer numerous benefits:

a. Remote Monitoring and Consultations

Telemedicine enables individuals to remotely monitor their glucose levels, share data with healthcare providers, and have virtual consultations.

This improves access to care, especially for individuals in remote areas or with mobility challenges.

b. Mobile Apps and Wearable Devices

Mobile applications and wearable devices provide tools for self-management, including glucose tracking, dietary guidance, physical activity monitoring, and medication reminders.

These technologies empower individuals to actively participate in their care and make informed decisions.

c. Behavioral Support and Coaching

Digital health solutions often incorporate behavioral support and coaching features to help individuals adopt and sustain healthy lifestyle habits.

These tools provide educational resources, goal-setting, and personalized feedback, promoting long-term behavior change.

6. Novel Drug Therapies

In addition to the established classes of glucose-lowering medications, ongoing research has identified novel drug therapies with the potential to revolutionize glucose management and cardiovascular health.

Some noteworthy developments include:

a. Glucagon-like Peptide-1 (GLP-1) Analogues

GLP-1 analogs are injectable medications that mimic the action of the hormone GLP-1.

These medications not only improve glucose control but have also shown cardiovascular benefits.

They reduce the risk of major adverse cardiovascular events, including heart attacks, strokes, and cardiovascular mortality.

GLP-1 analogs also promote weight loss and have positive effects on blood pressure and lipid profiles.

Sodium-Glucose Co-Transporter-2 (SGLT2) and Glucagon Receptor Antagonists: SGLT2 inhibitors have already been discussed as effective medications for glucose management and cardiovascular health.

However, ongoing research is exploring the potential of dual SGLT2 and glucagon receptor antagonists. These medications not only lower blood glucose levels but also suppress glucagon secretion, leading to improved glucose control and potential cardiovascular benefits.

Novel Insulin Formulations: Advancements in insulin formulations aim to enhance convenience, effectiveness, and safety.

Researchers are exploring ultra-rapid-acting insulin that mimic the physiological insulin response more closely, resulting in improved postprandial glucose control.

Furthermore, long-acting insulin with an extended duration of action and reduced risk of hypoglycemia are being developed to provide stable basal insulin coverage.

7. Gene Therapy

Gene therapy holds immense potential in the fields of glucose management and cardiovascular health.

It involves the delivery of specific genes to target cells to correct genetic defects or modify cellular functions.

While still in the early stages of development, gene therapy research is exploring avenues such as:

a. Genetic Editing of Beta Cells

Scientists are investigating methods to edit the genes of beta cells to enhance their insulin production and secretion capabilities.

This approach could lead to the restoration of normal glucose metabolism in individuals with diabetes.

b. Targeting Genetic Risk Factors

Gene therapy may also focus on targeting specific genetic risk factors associated with disturbances in glucose metabolism and cardiovascular disease.

By modifying these genetic factors, researchers hope to reduce the risk of developing these conditions.

c. Vascular Gene Therapy

Another potential application of gene therapy is targeting genes involved in blood vessel function and repair.

This could help improve vascular health and reduce the risk of cardiovascular complications associated with disturbances in glucose metabolism.

8. Artificial Intelligence and Machine Learning

Artificial intelligence (AI) and machine learning algorithms are being increasingly utilized in the fields of glucose management and cardiovascular health.

These technologies can analyze large datasets, identify patterns, and provide personalized recommendations.

Some applications include:

a. Predictive Analytics

AI algorithms can analyze patient data, including glucose levels, medication usage, lifestyle factors, and cardiovascular risk markers, to predict future health outcomes.

This can assist healthcare providers in proactively managing glucose control and cardiovascular risks.

b. Decision Support Systems

AI-powered decision support systems can help healthcare providers select the most appropriate treatment strategies based on individual patient characteristics, such as comorbidities, medication profiles, and cardiovascular risk factors.

These systems can assist in personalized treatment planning.

c. Wearable Technology Integration

AI algorithms can integrate with wearable devices, such as continuous glucose monitors and activity trackers, to analyze real-time data and provide actionable insights.

This can enable individuals to make informed decisions regarding their glucose management and cardiovascular health.

This Chapter has delved into the exciting realm of emerging therapies in glucose management and cardiovascular health.

Precision medicine, continuous glucose monitoring, artificial pancreas systems, stem cell therapy, telemedicine, novel drug therapies, gene therapy, and AI-based approaches all hold immense promise for transforming the way we manage disturbances in glucose metabolism and cardiovascular disease.

These advancements have the potential to improve outcomes, enhance the patient experience, and reduce the burden of these conditions on individuals and healthcare systems.

However, further research, clinical trials, and regulatory approvals are needed to ensure their safety, efficacy, and widespread availability.

As the field continues to evolve, the integration of these emerging therapies with existing approaches holds the key to optimizing glucose control and cardiovascular health in the future.

Chapter six

Lifestyle Interventions for Glucose Management and Cardiovascular Health

These interventions encompass various aspects, including diet, physical activity, weight management, stress reduction, and tobacco cessation.

By adopting a comprehensive and personalized approach, individuals can make meaningful changes that positively impact their health.

1-Dietary Modifications

Dietary choices have a profound influence on glucose control and cardiovascular health.

Some key considerations include:

a. Macronutrient Composition

A balanced diet that includes an appropriate distribution of carbohydrates, proteins, and fats is essential.

The specific macronutrient composition may vary depending on individual factors such as age, weight, activity level, and glucose management goals.

b. Carbohydrate Quality

Emphasizing complex carbohydrates from whole grains, legumes, fruits, and vegetables is recommended.

These foods provide fiber, vitamins, and minerals while having a lower impact on blood glucose levels.

c. Glycemic Index

Understanding the glycemic index (GI) of foods can help individuals make informed choices.

Foods with a lower GI release glucose more slowly, leading to more stable blood glucose levels.

d. Dietary Patterns

Mediterranean, DASH (Dietary Approaches to Stop Hypertension), and plant-based diets have shown beneficial effects on glucose control and cardiovascular health.

These diets emphasize whole foods, lean proteins, healthy fats, and limited processed foods.

2. Regular Physical Activity

Physical activity is vital for glucose management and cardiovascular health.

Regular exercise offers numerous benefits.

a. Glucose Control

Physical activity helps improve insulin sensitivity by facilitating glucose uptake by muscles and reducing insulin resistance.

This leads to better glucose control and a decreased risk of developing diabetes.

b. Weight Management

Engaging in regular physical activity aids in weight loss or maintenance, which is crucial for individuals with disturbances in glucose metabolism.

Maintaining a healthy weight improves insulin sensitivity and reduces cardiovascular risk.

c. Cardiovascular Health: Exercise strengthens the heart, improves circulation, lowers blood pressure, and increases high-density lipoprotein (HDL) cholesterol.

These factors collectively reduce the risk of cardiovascular disease.

d. Mental Well-being

Regular physical activity promotes mental well-being by reducing stress, anxiety, and depression.

Improved mental health positively impacts overall health and glucose management.

3. Weight Management

Maintaining a healthy weight is essential for optimizing glucose control and cardiovascular health.

Some strategies for weight management include:

a. Caloric Balance

Balancing energy intake and expenditure is crucial.

Consuming a moderate number of calories that align with individual needs and energy expenditure helps prevent weight gain.

b. Portion Control

Monitoring portion sizes can prevent overeating and promote weight management.

Understanding appropriate serving sizes and practicing mindful eating can support weight control.

c. Meal Planning

Planning meals and incorporating nutrient-dense foods, such as fruits, vegetables, lean proteins, and whole grains, can help individuals make healthier choices and manage weight effectively.

d. Behavior Modification

Adopting sustainable behavior changes, such as mindful eating, stress reduction techniques, and self-monitoring, can assist in long-term weight management.

4. Stress Reduction

Chronic stress can have negative effects on glucose control and cardiovascular health.

Implementing stress reduction techniques is beneficial.

a. Relaxation Techniques

Engaging in activities such as deep breathing exercises, meditation, yoga, and tai chi can help reduce stress levels and promote relaxation.

b. Adequate Sleep

Prioritizing quality sleep is crucial for stress management and overall health.

Sleep deprivation can affect glucose metabolism and increase cardiovascular risks.

c. Time Management

Effective time management strategies help individuals balance work, personal life, and self-care.

This can reduce stress levels and promote healthier lifestyle choices.

5. Tobacco Cessation

Smoking and tobacco use have detrimental effects on both glucose control and cardiovascular health.

Quitting tobacco offers significant benefits:

a. Reduced Cardiovascular Risks

Smoking increases the risk of heart disease, stroke, peripheral artery disease, and other cardiovascular conditions, quitting smoking can reverse some of these risks.

b. Improved Glucose Control

Smoking has been linked to insulin resistance and impaired glucose metabolism. Quitting smoking can improve insulin sensitivity and overall glucose control.

c. Overall Health Improvement

Smoking cessation has a positive impact on overall health, including respiratory function, immune system function, and reducing the risk of various cancers.

6. Behavioral Strategies for Sustainable Change

Adopting and maintaining lifestyle interventions requires behavioral strategies to facilitate sustainable change.

Some effective strategies include:

a. Goal Setting

Setting specific, measurable, attainable, relevant, and time-bound (SMART) goals helps individuals focus on their desired outcomes.

Breaking larger goals into smaller, more achievable steps increases motivation and success.

b. Self-Monitoring

Keeping track of behaviors, such as food intake, physical activity, and stress levels, through journals, mobile apps, or wearable devices enhances self-awareness.

This self-monitoring allows individuals to identify patterns, make adjustments, and stay accountable.

c. Social Support

Engaging in peer support groups, counseling, or involving family and friends in lifestyle changes can provide emotional support, encouragement, and accountability.

Social support networks offer motivation and a sense of community, fostering long-term adherence.

d. Cognitive Restructuring

Identifying and challenging negative thoughts and beliefs that hinder behavior change is important.

Replacing self-limiting beliefs with positive, empowering thoughts promotes self-efficacy and resilience.

e. Environmental Modification

Creating an environment that supports healthy choices can facilitate behavior change.

This includes removing temptations, stocking nutritious foods, making physical activity accessible, and reducing stress triggers in the environment.

7. Culturally Tailored Approaches

Recognizing and respecting individual cultural backgrounds is essential for successful lifestyle interventions.

Cultural factors influence dietary preferences, physical activity habits, and perceptions of health; tailoring interventions to align with cultural norms and values increases engagement and adherence.

Working collaboratively with individuals to incorporate culturally appropriate foods, activities, and traditions enhances the effectiveness and sustainability of lifestyle interventions.

8. Continuum of Care

Optimizing glucose management and cardiovascular health requires a continuum of care.

It involves ongoing monitoring, education, and support to ensure individuals maintain healthy lifestyle habits.

Key components of the continuum of care include:

a. Regular Follow-up

Periodic appointments with healthcare providers allow for monitoring progress, adjusting treatment plans, and addressing any challenges or concerns.

This ensures that individuals receive the necessary guidance and support.

b. Education and Empowerment

Providing comprehensive education on nutrition, physical activity, stress management, and self-care empowers individuals to make informed decisions and take ownership of their health.

Education can take various forms, including individual counseling, group sessions, workshops, or online resources.

c. Multidisciplinary Approach

Collaborating with a multidisciplinary team, including healthcare providers, dietitians, exercise specialists, psychologists, and pharmacists, ensures comprehensive and personalized care.

This team approach addresses the diverse needs and complexities of glucose management and cardiovascular health.

d. Long-term Support

Offering ongoing support, such as coaching, counseling, or access to support groups, helps individuals sustain lifestyle changes.

This support can be provided in person, through telemedicine, or via digital platforms.

This Chapter has highlighted the importance of lifestyle interventions in optimizing glucose management and cardiovascular health.

By implementing dietary modifications, engaging in regular physical activity, managing weight, reducing stress, quitting tobacco, and utilizing behavioral strategies, individuals can make sustainable changes that positively impact their health outcomes.

Incorporating culturally tailored approaches and ensuring a continuum of care enhances the effectiveness and long-term success of these interventions.

Healthcare providers play a pivotal role in guiding and supporting individuals throughout their journey toward improved glucose control, reduced cardiovascular risks, and enhanced overall well-being.

Through a comprehensive approach that combines medical interventions and lifestyle modifications, individuals can achieve lasting improvements in their glucose metabolism and cardiovascular health.

Chapter Seven

Technology and Digital Solutions for Glucose Management and Cardiovascular Health

Chapter seven explores the role of technology in optimizing glucose control, reducing cardiovascular risks, and improving overall health outcomes.

From glucose monitoring devices to mobile applications and telemedicine, these digital solutions offer convenience, personalized care, and enhanced patient engagement.

1. Continuous Glucose Monitoring (CGM) Systems

Continuous Glucose Monitoring (CGM) systems have revolutionized glucose management by providing real-time, dynamic data on glucose levels.

These systems consist of a small sensor placed under the skin that measures interstitial glucose levels and transmits data wirelessly to a receiver or smartphone app.

Key benefits of CGM systems include:

a. Real-time Feedback

CGM systems provide continuous and immediate feedback on glucose levels, allowing individuals to make timely adjustments to their medication, diet, and physical activity.

b. Trend Analysis

CGM systems display trends and patterns in glucose levels, highlighting high and low glucose excursions.

This information helps individuals and healthcare providers identify patterns, detect trends, and adjust treatment plans accordingly.

c. Alerts and Alarms

CGM systems can be programmed to provide alerts and alarms for hypoglycemia (low blood sugar) and hyperglycemia (high blood sugar).

These alerts prompt individuals to take appropriate actions, improving safety and preventing severe glucose fluctuations.

d. Data Sharing

Many CGM systems allow for data sharing with healthcare providers or family members.

This enables remote monitoring and enhances communication, ensuring timely interventions and support.

2. Insulin Pump Therapy

Insulin pump therapy offers an alternative to multiple daily injections for individuals with diabetes.

These small devices deliver a continuous supply of rapid-acting insulin subcutaneously.

Key advantages of insulin pump therapy include:

a. Basal Rate Adjustment

Insulin pumps allow for personalized basal rate adjustments, mimicking physiological insulin secretion more closely.

This customization enables tighter glucose control and flexibility in managing daily activities and variable insulin requirements.

b. Bolus Dose Calculation

Insulin pumps offer precise bolus dose calculations based on carbohydrate intake, current glucose levels, and individual insulin sensitivity.

This feature simplifies insulin dosing and improves postprandial glucose control.

c. Data Logging

Insulin pumps often have built-in glucose monitoring capabilities or can be integrated with CGM systems.

This data-logging feature provides a comprehensive overview of glucose levels, insulin doses, and trends, aiding in therapy adjustments and treatment optimization.

d. Connectivity

Many insulin pumps can be connected to smartphone apps or computer software, allowing for remote monitoring and data sharing with healthcare providers.

This connectivity streamlines communication, enhances remote management, and facilitates timely adjustments.

3. Mobile Applications (Apps)

Mobile applications have transformed glucose management and cardiovascular health.

These apps offer various functionalities, including:

a. Glucose Tracking

Mobile apps enable individuals to log and track their glucose levels, medication usage, and meals.

This feature provides a comprehensive overview of glucose control and supports self-management.

b. Meal Planning and Nutrition Tracking

Some apps offer meal planning features, providing access to nutritional information, carbohydrate counting tools, and recipe ideas.

This supports individuals in making informed dietary choices and optimizing glucose control.

c. Physical Activity Monitoring

Many apps include physical activity tracking features, allowing individuals to monitor their exercise routines, set activity goals, and track progress.

This promotes regular physical activity and aids in weight management.

d. Medication Reminders

Apps can send medication reminders and notifications to help individuals adhere to their medication schedules, improving treatment compliance and glucose control.

4. Telemedicine

Telemedicine, the use of telecommunications technology for remote healthcare consultations, has gained significant prominence.

Key aspects of telemedicine for glucose management and cardiovascular health include:

a. Remote Consultations

Telemedicine enables individuals to have virtual consultations with healthcare providers from the comfort of their homes.

This eliminates the need for travel, reduces barriers to access, and improves convenience.

b. Glucose Monitoring and Remote Data Analysis

Individuals can transmit glucose data from their devices, such as CGM systems or glucometers, to healthcare providers.

This allows for remote monitoring, data analysis, and treatment adjustments based on real-time information.

c. Education and Support

Telemedicine platforms facilitate educational sessions, counseling and support groups through virtual means.

This enhances patient education, self-management skills, and emotional support.

d. Follow-up Care

Telemedicine allows for regular follow-up visits and continuous care.

Healthcare providers can monitor progress, address concerns, and provide ongoing guidance, ensuring that individuals receive the necessary support and adjustments to their treatment plans.

5. Artificial Intelligence (AI) and Machine Learning

Artificial Intelligence (AI) and Machine Learning algorithms have shown promising applications in glucose management and cardiovascular health.

These technologies can analyze vast amounts of data, identify patterns, and provide personalized recommendations.

Key applications include:

a. Glucose Prediction

AI algorithms can analyze historical glucose data, along with factors such as food intake, physical activity, and medication usage, to predict future glucose levels.

This predictive capability helps individuals proactively manage their glucose control and prevent extreme fluctuations.

b. Decision Support Systems

AI-powered decision support systems can provide personalized treatment recommendations based on individual characteristics, glucose patterns, and cardiovascular risk factors.

These systems help healthcare providers make informed decisions and optimize treatment plans.

c. Risk Stratification

Machine Learning algorithms can analyze patient data, including medical history, demographics, and laboratory results, to identify individuals at high risk of developing cardiovascular complications.

This risk stratification enables early intervention and targeted preventive measures.

d. Personalized Interventions

AI algorithms can provide personalized recommendations for dietary modifications, physical activity goals, and medication adjustments based on individual preferences, goals, and response patterns.

This tailoring improves patient engagement and adherence to recommended interventions.

6. Wearable Devices

Wearable devices have gained popularity for their ability to monitor various health parameters and promote an active lifestyle.

Some key wearable devices include:

a. Fitness Trackers

These devices monitor physical activity, such as steps taken, distance traveled, and calories burned.

They provide individuals with real-time feedback, encouraging them to maintain an active lifestyle and achieve their physical activity goals.

b. Smart watches

Smart watches offer features like heart rate monitoring, sleep tracking, and activity reminders.

These devices provide insights into cardiovascular health, stress levels, and overall well-being, aiding individuals in making healthier choices.

c. Blood Pressure Monitors

Wearable blood pressure monitors allow individuals to track their blood pressure trends and share the data with healthcare providers.

This promotes proactive management of hypertension and reduces the risk of cardiovascular complications.

d. Glucometers and CGM Integration

Some wearable devices integrate glucose monitoring capabilities, enabling continuous glucose monitoring or on-demand blood glucose measurements.

This integration enhances convenience and simplifies glucose management for individuals.

7. Data Privacy and Security

With the increasing use of technology in healthcare, ensuring data privacy and security is of utmost importance.

Protecting personal health information and maintaining data integrity are critical considerations.

It is essential to

a. Implement Secure Data Transmission

Encryption and secure data transmission protocols should be employed to protect patient data during transmission between devices, apps, and healthcare providers.

b. Secure Data Storage

Robust measures must be in place to safeguard stored patient data, including secure servers, access controls, and data backup systems.

Compliance with data protection regulations, such as HIPAA, is crucial.

c. User Consent and Control

Individuals should have control over their data, including the ability to provide informed consent for data sharing, access, and usage. Transparent privacy policies and clear communication are necessary to maintain trust and respect patient autonomy.

d. Cyber security Measures

Healthcare systems and devices should be protected against cyber threats, including malware, hacking, and unauthorized access.

Regular security assessments, software updates, and employee training are vital to maintaining cyber security.

This Chapter has explored the use of technology and digital solutions in glucose management and cardiovascular health.

From Artificial Intelligence (AI) and Machine Learning algorithms to wearable devices and data privacy considerations, these advancements have the potential to revolutionize healthcare delivery.

By leveraging technology, individuals can monitor their glucose levels, receive personalized recommendations, and actively participate in their care.

However, it is crucial to prioritize data privacy, security, and ethical considerations to ensure responsible.

Chapter Eight

Integrative Approaches for Glucose Management and Cardiovascular Health

ntegrative medicine combines conventional medical interventions with evidence-based complementary therapies, emphasizing the whole person and addressing the interconnectedness of physical, mental, emotional, and spiritual aspects of health.

This chapter explores various integrative approaches and their potential benefits in promoting well-being and managing disturbances in glucose metabolism and cardiovascular health.

1. Mind-Body Techniques

Mind-body techniques encompass practices that emphasize the connection between the mind, emotions, and physical health.

These techniques promote relaxation, stress reduction, and overall well-being.

Key mind-body techniques include:

a. Meditation

 Meditation involves focusing attention and achieving a state of deep relaxation and mental clarity.

Regular meditation practice has been shown to reduce stress, improve emotional well-being, and enhance glucose control.

b. Yoga

Yoga combines physical postures, breathing exercises, and meditation to promote physical and mental well-being.

Yoga has demonstrated positive effects on glucose metabolism, cardiovascular health, stress reduction, and flexibility.

c. Tai Chi

Tai Chi is a gentle, low-impact exercise that involves slow, flowing movements and deep breathing.

Practicing Tai Chi has been associated with improved glucose control, reduced cardiovascular risks, enhanced balance, and increased overall vitality.

d. Biofeedback

Biofeedback techniques involve using devices to monitor and provide real-time feedback on physiological parameters, such as heart rate, blood pressure, and muscle tension.

By learning to regulate these functions, individuals can enhance their self-awareness and self-regulation abilities.

2. Nutritional and Herbal Interventions

Nutritional and herbal interventions can complement conventional treatments in optimizing glucose control and cardiovascular health.

Some key approaches include:

a. Medical Nutrition Therapy (MNT)

MNT involves individualized nutrition counseling and education to promote healthy eating habits and manage glucose levels.

It focuses on carbohydrate counting, portion control, and balanced meal planning.

b. Dietary Supplements

Certain dietary supplements, such as omega-3 fatty acids, chromium, cinnamon, and berberine, have shown potential for improving glucose control and reducing cardiovascular risks.

However, it is important to consult healthcare providers before starting any supplements, as they may interact with medications or have potential side effects.

c. Herbal Medicine

Herbal remedies, such as ginseng, bitter melon, fenugreek, and cinnamon, have been traditionally used to support glucose control.

While some herbs may have potential benefits, their use should be approached with caution, and consultation with a qualified herbalist or healthcare provider is recommended.

d. Functional Foods

 Functional foods are those that provide additional
health benefits beyond basic nutrition.

Incorporating foods like whole grains, legumes, fruits,
vegetables, and probiotics into the diet can support
glucose management, cardiovascular health, and overall
well-being.

3. Acupuncture

Acupuncture is an ancient Chinese therapy that involves
inserting thin needles at specific points in the body to
stimulate physiological responses.

Acupuncture has been shown to have potential benefits
for glucose control and cardiovascular health by:

a. Regulating Hormones

 Acupuncture may help regulate insulin levels, improve
insulin sensitivity, and modulate hormones involved in
glucose metabolism.

b. Reducing Inflammation

Acupuncture has anti-inflammatory effects that may help reduce systemic inflammation, which is associated with insulin resistance and cardiovascular risks.

c. Enhancing Circulation

Acupuncture has been found to improve blood circulation, which can support cardiovascular health and tissue healing.

d. Stress Reduction

Acupuncture promotes relaxation and can help reduce stress, which is beneficial for overall health and glucose control.

4. Mindful Eating

Mindful eating involves paying attention to the sensory experiences, thoughts, and emotions associated with eating.

By cultivating awareness and making conscious food choices, mindful eating can support glucose management and cardiovascular health by:

a. Enhancing Food Awareness

 Mindful eating helps individuals become more aware of their food choices, portion sizes, and hunger and fullness cues.

This can lead to more balanced and mindful eating habits.

b. Promoting Satiety

 Mindful eating encourages individuals to eat slowly, savoring each bite, and paying attention to feelings of fullness.

This can prevent overeating and support healthy weight management.

c. Emotional Regulation

Mindful eating helps individuals recognize emotional trigger for eating and develop alternative coping strategies, reducing emotional eating and promoting a healthier relationship with food.

d. Conscious Food Choices

Mindful eating encourages individuals to choose foods that nourish their bodies, focusing on nutrient-dense options and Mindful indulgences rather than restrictive or impulsive eating patterns.

5. Physical Activity and Exercise

Physical activity and exercise play a crucial role in maintaining glucose control and cardiovascular health.

Regular exercise has numerous benefits, including:

a. Improved Insulin Sensitivity

Exercise helps improve insulin sensitivity, allowing cells to better utilize glucose and reducing the risk of insulin resistance.

b. Weight Management

Physical activity contributes to weight management by burnin calories and promoting lean muscle mass.

Maintaining a healthy weight is important for glucose control and cardiovascular health.

c. Cardiovascular Fitness

Exercise strengthens the heart and improves cardiovascular fitness.

It can help reduce blood pressure, lower LDL cholesterol levels, and enhance overall cardiovascular health.

d. Stress Reduction

 Engaging in physical activity can reduce stress levels, which can have a positive impact on glucose control and cardiovascular health.

It is important to note that individuals should consult with their healthcare providers before starting any exercise regimen, especially if they have pre-existing health conditions or are new to exercise.

6. Sleep and Stress Management

Adequate sleep and effective stress management are essential components of glucose management and cardiovascular health.

Poor sleep and chronic stress can negatively impact glucose control and increase the risk of cardiovascular complications.

Key considerations include:

a. Sleep Hygiene

Practicing good sleep hygiene involves adopting habits that promote quality sleep, such as maintaining a consistent sleep schedule, creating a conducive sleep environment, and avoiding stimulants before bedtime.

b. Stress Reduction Techniques

Managing stress is crucial for overall well-being,

Techniques such as deep breathing exercises, meditation, mindfulness practices, and engaging in hobbies or activities that bring joy and relaxation can help reduce stress levels and improve glucose control.

c. Cognitive Behavioral Therapy (CBT)

CBT is a therapeutic approach that focuses on identifying and modifying negative thought patterns and behaviors.

It can be beneficial for managing stress, improving sleep, and supporting overall mental well-being.

d. Relaxation Techniques

Incorporating relaxation techniques such as progressive muscle relaxation, guided imagery, and aromatherapy can help individuals unwind, reduce stress, and promote better sleep.

7. Social Support and Community Engagement

Social support and community engagement play a vital role in glucose management and cardiovascular health.

Connecting with others who share similar health goals can provide motivation, emotional support, and practical assistance.

Some strategies to foster social support and community engagement include:

a. Support Groups

Joining support groups or online communities focused on glucose management and cardiovascular health can provide a platform for sharing experiences, exchanging knowledge, and receiving emotional support.

b. Healthcare Team Collaboration

Building a collaborative relationship with healthcare provider ensures ongoing support and guidance in managing glucose levels and cardiovascular health.

Regular checkups and open communication are crucial.

c. Lifestyle Interventions

Engaging in group-based lifestyle interventions, such as exercise classes, cooking workshops, or diabetes self-management programs, can foster a sense of community and accountability while promoting healthy behaviors.

d. Family and Friends

Informing family and friends about glucose management and cardiovascular health goals can garner support and understanding.

Engaging in activities together, such as cooking healthy meals or participating in physical activities, can strengthen bonds while promoting a healthy lifestyle.

This Chapter has explored integrative approaches for optimizing glucose management and cardiovascular health.

Mind-body techniques, nutritional interventions, acupuncture, mindful eating, physical activity, sleep and stress management, and social support are all essential components of a holistic approach.

By integrating these approaches, individuals can enhance their overall well-being, improve glucose control, reduce cardiovascular risks, and enjoy a higher quality of life.

It is important to personalize these approaches based on individual needs and preferences while seeking guidance from qualified healthcare providers.

The integration of these integrative approaches with conventional care can provide a comprehensive and well-rounded approach to glucose management and cardiovascular health, empowering individuals to take control of their health and well-being.

Chapter Nine

Behavioral Strategies for Sustaining Healthy Glucose Management and Cardiovascular Health

While medical interventions and lifestyle changes are crucial, long-term success relies on cultivating positive behaviors and habits.

This chapter explores various behavioral strategies that individuals can employ to support their glucose control and cardiovascular well-being.

1. Goal Setting

Setting clear and achievable goals is an essential behavioral strategy for sustaining healthy glucose management and cardiovascular health.

Key considerations for effective goal setting include:

a. Specificity

Goals should be specific, measurable, and time-bound.

For example, rather than setting a goal to "exercise more," it is more effective to set a goal of "walking for 30 minutes five days a week."

b. Realistic and Attainable

Goals should be realistic and attainable based on individual capabilities, resources, and lifestyle factors.

Setting overly ambitious goals can lead to frustration and demotivation.

c. Personalization

Goals should be personalized to individual preferences and needs.

Taking personal interests, preferences, and motivations into account increases the likelihood of adherence and success.

d. Monitoring Progress

Regularly monitoring and tracking progress toward goals provides feedback and motivation.

This can be done through self-monitoring tools such as glucose logs, activity trackers, or journaling.

2. Self-Monitoring

Self-monitoring involves actively tracking and recording behaviors, physiological parameters, and outcomes related to glucose management and cardiovascular health.

Key aspects of self-monitoring include:

a. Glucose Monitoring

Regularly monitoring blood glucose levels, whether through self-monitoring devices or continuous glucose monitoring systems, provides valuable information for making informed decisions about diet, medication, and physical activity.

b. Food and Beverage Intake

Keeping a food diary or using mobile apps to track food and beverage intake helps individuals become aware of their dietary patterns, identify triggers for glucose fluctuations, and make necessary adjustments.

c. Physical Activity Tracking

Using wearable devices or smartphone apps to monitor physical activity levels, steps taken, and exercise duration can promote awareness and accountability.

d. Emotions and Stress Levels

 Tracking emotions, stress levels, and their potential impact on glucose control can help individuals identify patterns and implement strategies for stress reduction and emotional well-being.

3. Cognitive Behavioral Therapy (CBT)

Cognitive Behavioral Therapy (CBT) is a therapeutic approach that focuses on identifying and modifying negative thought patterns and behaviors.

CBT can be valuable in supporting healthy glucose management and cardiovascular health by:

a. Identifying Cognitive Distortions

 CBT helps individuals recognize and challenge cognitive distortions, such as negative self-talk, catastrophizing, or all-or-nothing thinking, that may hinder healthy behaviors.

b. Behavior Modification

CBT assists individuals in identifying and modifying behaviors that contribute to poor glucose control or cardiovascular risks, such as emotional eating, sedentary habits, or non-adherence to medication regimens.

c. Stress Management

CBT equips individuals with stress management techniques, such as relaxation exercises, problem-solving skills, and cognitive restructuring, to cope effectively with stressors that impact glucose management and cardiovascular health.

d. Motivation Enhancement

CBT can enhance motivation and promote behavior change by identifying and reinforcing intrinsic motivators, setting realistic goals, and addressing potential barriers to change.

4. Social Support and Accountability

Social support and accountability play vital roles in sustaining healthy behaviors and promoting glucose control and cardiovascular well-being.

Strategies to harness social support include

a. Informing Loved Ones

Sharing glucose management and cardiovascular health goals with family, friends, and close contacts can provide support, encouragement, and understanding.

b. Supportive Networks

Joining support groups, online communities, or wellness programs focused on glucose management and cardiovascular health can provide opportunities for information sharing, mutual support, and accountability.

c. Partnered Approach

 Engaging in healthy behaviors together with a partner or loved one can create a supportive environment and increase the likelihood of adherence to healthy habits.

d. Healthcare Provider Collaboration

 Collaborating closely with healthcare providers ensures ongoing support, guidance, and accountability in maintaining healthy behaviors and managing glucose and cardiovascular health.

5. Motivational Interviewing

Motivational Interviewing (MI) is a counseling approach that focuses on enhancing an individual's motivation and commitment to behavior change.

MI can be beneficial for sustaining healthy glucose management and cardiovascular health by:

a. Exploring Ambivalence

 MI helps individuals explore and resolve any ambivalence or conflicting feelings they may have about making behavior changes.

This allows for a deeper understanding of their motivations and barriers to change.

b. Enhancing Intrinsic Motivation

 MI encourages individuals to identify and connect with their intrinsic motivations for adopting and maintaining healthy behaviors.

By exploring personal values, goals, and aspirations, individuals can strengthen their commitment to behavior change.

c. Supporting Autonomy

 MI emphasizes the individual's autonomy and decision-making abilities, fostering a sense of empowerment and ownership over their health choices.

This approach respects individual preferences and values, increasing the likelihood of sustained behavior change.

d. Building Self-Efficacy

 MI helps individuals identify and build confidence in their ability to make and sustain behavior changes.

By exploring past successes and developing a plan for overcoming obstacles, individuals can increase their self-efficacy and belief in their ability to manage glucose and cardiovascular health.

6. Environmental Modification

Modifying the environment can have a significant impact on sustaining healthy behaviors related to glucose management and cardiovascular health.

Consider the following strategies:

a. Creating a Supportive Home Environment

Ensure the home environment is conducive to healthy behaviors, such as having a well-stocked kitchen with nutritious foods, creating a designated exercise area, and removing triggers for unhealthy habits.

b. Workplace Support

Advocate for supportive policies and practices in the workplace that promote healthy behaviors, such as access to healthy food options, standing or walking breaks, and wellness programs.

c. Accessibility and Convenience

Make healthy choices more accessible and convenient by arranging the physical environment to support these behaviors.

For example, placing fruits and vegetables at eye level in the refrigerator or keeping exercise equipment visible and easily accessible

d. Social Norms

Cultivate social norms that promote and support healthy behaviors.

Encourage friends, family, and coworkers to engage in activities that prioritize glucose management and cardiovascular health, such as group exercise sessions or healthy potluck meals.

7. Continuous Learning and Adaptation

Sustaining healthy behaviors requires ongoing learning, adaptation, and refinement of strategies.

Individuals should consider:

a. Staying Informed

Stay up-to-date with current research, guidelines, and advancements in glucose management and cardiovascular health.

This knowledge can inform decision-making and provide new strategies to incorporate into daily routines.

b. Regular Evaluation

Regularly evaluate progress toward goals, reassess behaviors, and identify areas for improvement.

This self-reflection allows individuals to make necessary adjustments and maintain a growth mindset.

c. Flexibility and Resilience

Recognize that setbacks and challenges are a natural part of behavior change.

Cultivate flexibility and resilience to bounce back from setbacks and adapt strategies when faced with obstacles.

d. Celebrating Milestones

Acknowledge and celebrate achievements along the journey.

Celebrating milestones, whether small or significant, reinforces positive behaviors and serves as a reminder of the progress made.

This Chapter has explored behavioral strategies for sustaining healthy glucose management and cardiovascular health.

Goal setting, self-monitoring, cognitive-behavioral techniques, social support, motivational interviewing, environmental modification, continuous learning, and adaptation are all crucial aspects of maintaining positive habits.

By incorporating these strategies into daily life, individuals can enhance their motivation, sustain healthy behaviors, and effectively manage their glucose and cardiovascular health in the long term.

It is important to personalize these strategies to individual needs and circumstances while seeking support from healthcare professionals or behavioral health specialists when necessary.

The integration of behavioral strategies with other interventions and lifestyle modifications forms a comprehensive approach to sustaining glucose management and cardiovascular well-being, empowering individuals to lead healthier and more fulfilling lives.

Chapter Ten

Strategies for Long-Term Maintenance and Preventing Relapse

Chapter 10 explores strategies for long-term maintenance and preventing relapse in glucose management and cardiovascular health.

Sustaining positive changes and preventing a return to unhealthy habits are crucial for achieving lasting benefits.

This chapter discusses various strategies that individuals can employ to maintain their progress and minimize the risk of relapse.

1- Continued Self-Monitoring

Continued self-monitoring plays a vital role in long-term maintenance.

Key aspects of self-monitoring include:

a. Regular Glucose Monitoring

Ongoing monitoring of blood glucose levels provides valuable feedback and enables individuals to make informed decisions about their diet, physical activity, and medication management.

b. Periodic Health Check-ups

Regular check-ups with healthcare providers allow for comprehensive assessment, monitoring of cardiovascular health, and adjustment of treatment plans as needed.

c. Tracking Behaviors

Continuing to track food intake, physical activity, and other relevant behaviors helps individuals stay accountable and maintain awareness of their habits.

d. Emotional Well-being Monitoring

Monitoring emotions and stress levels remain important, as emotional well-being can significantly impact glucose management and cardiovascular health.

2. Maintenance Goals

Setting and maintaining new goals is essential for long-term success.

Consider the following strategies:

a. Setting Long-Term Goals

Alongside short-term goals, establish long-term goals that reflect the desired lifestyle and outcomes in glucose management and cardiovascular health.

These goals can provide direction and motivation.

b. SMART Goals

Ensure goals are Specific, Measurable, Achievable, Relevant, and Time-bound. SMART goals increase the likelihood of success and help individuals track their progress effectively.

c. Gradual Progression

Continuously challenge yourself by gradually increasing the difficulty or intensity of goals.

This gradual progression helps avoid complacency and promotes continuous improvement.

d. Lifestyle Integration

Aim to integrate healthy behaviors into your daily life rather than considering them as short-term changes.

This shift in mindset supports long-term maintenance.

3. Positive Reinforcement

Applying positive reinforcement techniques can help reinforce and maintain healthy behaviors.

Consider these strategies:

a. Celebrating Achievements

Acknowledge and celebrate milestones along the journey.

Rewarding yourself for reaching goals or sustaining healthy habits can boost motivation and reinforce positive behaviors.

b. Self-Reflection

Regularly reflect on the positive changes and benefits experienced due to improved glucose management and cardiovascular health.

This self-reflection reinforces the value of maintaining healthy habits.

c. Social Support

Engage with a supportive network of family, friends, or support groups who can provide encouragement, validation, and reinforcement of healthy behaviors.

d. Intrinsic Motivation

Cultivate intrinsic motivation by connecting with the personal values and reasons behind your desire to maintain glucose control and cardiovascular health.

Remind yourself of the intrinsic rewards and benefits gained from these behaviors.

4. Coping with Setbacks

Setbacks are a natural part of the journey, but it's important to develop effective coping strategies:

a. Resilience Building

Cultivate resilience by recognizing setbacks as learning opportunities rather than failures.

Embrace a growth mindset that allows for adjustments and continued progress.

b. Problem Solving Skills

Develop problem-solving skills to overcome challenges and barriers that may arise. Identify potential obstacles and strategize ways to address them effectively.

c. Seek Support

Reach out to healthcare providers, counselors, or support networks for guidance and assistance when facing difficulties or experiencing a relapse.

Utilizing the available support systems a help get back on track.

d. Self-Compassion

Practice self-compassion during setbacks or relapses.

Be kind to yourself, acknowledge the challenges faced, and recommit to the desired behaviors and habits.

5. Lifestyle Integration

Integration of healthy behaviors into daily life is a key strategy for long-term maintenance.

Consider the following approaches:

a. Habit Formation

Focus on developing healthy habits that become automatic over time.

Consistently engaging in healthy behaviors, such as regular exercise, balanced nutrition, and medication adherence, helps embed these habits into daily routines.

b. Environmental Cues

Create an environment that supports healthy choices.

For example, keep healthy snacks readily available, set reminders for medication intake, or establish a designated exercise space at home.

c. Mindful Decision-Making

Practice mindful decision-making by considering the long-term consequences of choices.

When faced with decisions related to food, physical activity, or stress management, consciously choose options that align with glucose management and cardiovascular health goals.

d. Sustainable Approach

Strive for a sustainable approach to lifestyle changes.

Avoid extreme or restrictive behaviors that are difficult to maintain in the long term.

Instead, focus on making gradual, realistic changes that can be sustained over time.

6. Social Support and Accountability

Continued social support and accountability contribute to long-term maintenance.

Consider the following strategies:

a. Supportive Relationships

Surround yourself with individuals who support and encourage your efforts in glucose management and cardiovascular health.

Engage in open communication with loved ones, sharing challenges, and seeking their understanding and assistance.

b. Supportive Programs

Participate in structured programs or support groups that offer ongoing support and guidance.

These platforms provide opportunities for learning, sharing experiences, and holding each other accountable.

c. Buddy System

Find an accountability partner or exercise buddy who shares similar goals.

Having someone to engage in healthy activities with and hold each other accountable can increase motivation and commitment.

d. Virtual Communities

Utilize online communities, forums, or social media groups focused on glucose management and cardiovascular health.

These platforms provide a space for knowledge-sharing, motivation, and support from like-minded individuals.

7. Maintenance Planning

Developing a maintenance plan ensures preparedness for potential challenges and helps prevent relapse.

Consider the following aspects:

a. Anticipating Triggers

Identify potential triggers or high-risk situations that may lead to relapse.

This could include stress, social events, or travel. Develop strategies to cope with these triggers effectively and maintain healthy behaviors.

b. Relapse Prevention Techniques

Learn relapse prevention techniques, such as identifying early warning signs, developing coping strategies, and engaging in alternative activities to prevent a return to unhealthy habits.

c. Revisiting Strategies

Regularly review and refine the strategies that have been effective for you.

Adapt and modify approaches as needed to ensure they remain relevant and supportive of your glucose management and cardiovascular health goals.

d. Long-Term Vision

 Maintain a clear vision of your long-term health goals.

Remind yourself of the benefits and reasons behind your desire to maintain glucose control and cardiovascular health.

This vision can serve as a powerful motivator in times of temptation or difficulty.

This Chapter has discussed strategies for long-term maintenance and preventing relapse in glucose management and cardiovascular health.

By continuing self-monitoring, setting maintenance goals, utilizing positive reinforcement, coping with setbacks, integrating healthy behaviors into daily life, seeking social support and accountability, and developing a maintenance plan, individuals can sustain their progress and minimize the risk of relapse.

It is important to personalize these strategies based on individual needs, preferences, and circumstances.

Remember that maintenance is an ongoing process, and with dedication, perseverance, and a comprehensive approach, individuals can enjoy the benefits of improved glucose management and cardiovascular health for years to come.